MW01226964

Sex Life after 60

(Common Issues to Consider if you want to have a Great Sex Life after 60)

Haytham Al Fiqi

ISBN-13:978-1523940394

ISBN-10:1523940395

DEDICATION

This book of the best designed books that can be read and benefit from your life in general

ACKNOWLEDGMENTS

All thanks and appreciation to those who helped me with this book

1- Common Issues to Consider if you want to have a Great Sex Life after 60

Some individuals really have a fear of getting older. They don't want to be viewed by society as a has been. They aren't really sure what their future holds so they tend to dwell on it. They may have memories of their own parents or grandparents with difficulties as they got older. It is only natural not to want to follow along that same path.

If you want to have a great sex life after the age of 60 then you need to really think about it now. What is your current sex life like? Do you enjoy the activity or do you just go through the motions? Are you in a serious and committed relationship that you would definitely like to still be involved in when that time comes?

Some people in their 30's and even their 40's put sex on the back burner. That is understandable with all of the various commitments we often have in our lives. People are on the fast track and over committed. There are family issues, career, and trying to find some time for yourself. It can leave a person drained and with two people on different schedules it is even more difficult.

Many researchers will tell you that the type of sex life you have in your younger years will influence how it is for you after 60. So if you aren't happy with what you have now you need to make some changes. Finding ways to be very happy with your own sexuality is very important. The number of people who aren't sexually happy is very high, yet very few of them are willing to express what needs to change to their partners.

Part of the problem though is the attitude that earlier generations had about sex. Many women still feel that it is their duty to please their man. Therefore they don't talk openly about wanting more or less sex. They don't express their desires of what they want to see happen. Since no one is bringing it up, their partners just assume they are pleasing them.

If you find that your life is one I mentioned about being too full for sex, then you need to cut back. Make a commitment to make sex something that is important in your relationship. It shouldn't be the only thing you have going, but certainly a perk. If you and your partner are having to pencil each other in for sexual activities then changes need to be made sooner than later.

Some individuals over the age of 60 find that their living conditions can become an issue as well. You may be ready to go to some type of assisted living facility rather than to live on your own. Are they going to approve of sexual activities taking place there? It is important to know what those guidelines are. Some places such as nursing homes don't allow it and there certainly is very little privacy.

Even if you end up living with your adult children in your older years, are you going to be comfortable with sexual activities? Many adults don't want their children to know about it even though they aren't little kids any more. The issue is further compounded when the parent living with them is dating instead of actually married.

There are many common issues to consider if you want to have a great sex life after 60. The main focus needs to be on what is going to make you and your partner very happy. There is no reason though not to enjoy sex if it is something you find to be important. You may have some barriers to deal with along the way, but with some accurate information and openness you can find solutions to them that will work well for you.

2- Why Sex is Different for those over 60

Sex has a way of making relationships difficult when we are younger. Many young people struggle with the issue of when it is the right time for them to start having sex. They may feel they have found the right person and then down the road wish they had waited for someone else to share that experience with.

Many people will tell you that having sex at a young age can certainly lead to some difficulties with relationships. One party may want it to be very casual while the other has fallen in love. There are hurt feelings and even unwanted pregnancies that have to be dealt with. Some may say that they don't want to think about sex and being older, but those over 60 will tell you it is different – and the love it.

They don't have to deal with all the same struggles as they once did. Most women over 60 will tell you that they don't have to worry about looks. They know that the partner they are with wants to be with them for more than just the hot body they have. They have accepted that their body has changed with time and they still enjoy having sex.

Men over the age of 60 will also tell you that the burden is off them to have the big muscles. They also don't have to try to perform all night long like they did in their younger years. With all of the stress off the issue of having sex, the couple can focus on making each other feel good. It is a completely different feeling than what they experienced before.

Both sexes will agree that sex at this age is about much more than just the physical side of things. It is a way to connect with someone they love, respect, and desire on a deeper level. Sex doesn't have to be the central theme of the relationship so there isn't any pressure for it to start taking place. They can take their time to get to know each other before they move on to that level.

For couples who have been together for a very long time, they often find as they move into their 60's that they have more time to spend with each other. This allows them to rekindle their love for each other that may have been pushed aside for many of the past years in their relationship.

You will definitely find these types of relationships to be built on great communication. They two people will really enjoy being around each other. They love to talk and to spend time together. Having sex is just an added benefit of them spending that time with each other. They can bring that level of communication that they value into the sexual relationship as well.

For those over 60, still having sex means that someone finds you to be desirable. This is very important to both men and women. It allows them to feel loved and cared for. It also allows them to have a level of intimacy that goes beyond just sitting close or holding hands with someone. That can help them to feel young and revitalized.

You will also find that as people get older they value their relationships more. Even though young couples may be in love, they may not fully realize the importance of their choices. Older individuals are able to see the connection of a good relationship both outside of the bedroom and inside of it. That is what keeps their passion for each other alive.

If you fit into the category of individuals who think it isn't going to be much fun having sex one you are 60, think again. Re-evaluate your attitude about it once you have read the material online for those who are in that age group and loving their sex life. Things are going to change but having sex in your 60's and beyond can be a completely new experience. It can be more rewarding in many ways then what you experienced at earlier times in your life.

3- Tips for Enjoying a Healthy and Happy Sex Life into your 60's

The issue of older individuals having sex is becoming more common. Many believe this has to do with baby boomers out there that are more open to the topic. They don't find it to be as taboo as it once was. Also, women feel there is more equality in today's society than in the past. They are more open to talk about their sexual relationships instead of hiding them as they once did.

There is no reason to think you won't be able to enjoy a very healthy and happy sex life into your 60's as well. Keeping yourself feeling good now is very important regardless of what age you currently are at. If you aren't enjoying sex now in your 30's or 40's you need to be asking yourself why not. You need to be facing those issues so you can get better results from the activity.

It is important to have a commitment to your partner too. Both of you want to be able to continue enjoying sex into your 60's and beyond. It can be difficult when one of the people in the relationship isn't able to enjoy it or to perform. By looking out for the health of each other it is going to make it possible though.

You need to feel your very best if you want to enjoy sex at that age though. Getting enough rest and enough exercise is very important. Walking as a couple can allow you to have to time to visit and communicate. At the same time you will be promoting your health and a better sex life into the future.

Don't underestimate the value of eating right either. It can be great to try out new recipes that are good for you. Cooking as a couple can be fun and make it less of a chore. You will also find this keeps both of you healthy enough to continue enjoying sex as you are getting older.

If you don't have a partner when you enter your 60's you should be more receptive to the idea. Some individuals of that age group continue to be old fashioned. They aren't willing to have sex with someone until they are married. That is a different look than what today's society promotes. There is also the issue of protecting yourself against sexually transmitted diseases too when you are with a new partner.

Everyone should be seeing a doctor annually for a full check up. These appointments are essential as early intervention can help to prevent problems that lead to not enjoying sex. If you have any problems enjoying it before that annual exam is due then schedule another appointment. Your doctor can assist you with getting your sex life back to a place where you are happy with it once again.

It can take some patience in order to deal with problems along the way. There are many that affect both men and women. Being aware of the changes in your sexual behaviors is important. Be willing to talk about them with your partner so they know what you need. During the times when you can't enjoy sex, you can still enjoy other levels of intimacy with each other. This will help keep the passion alive and encourage the partner to seek the assistance they need.

Do your part to ensure you are able to enjoy a healthy and happy sex life into your 60's. There is no reason why that part of your life should stop because of your age. Staying active physically, staying connected emotionally, and even being social will all help you to really get the most out of it. Sex is a great way to share yourself with another person and you will likely want to continue doing so as you get older. Make sure you take measures now to ensure it is going to be a possibility for you.

4- Dealing with Changes in your Sexual Relationship when you are 60 or Older

There are going to be some changes in a person's life as they get older, there is nothing that can be done about it. One of them is that your sexual relationship is going to change. For some people it is for the better and for others it leaves them wishing for their younger days. Those that seem to enjoy sex more as they get older often find that with the reduction of stress in their life they can get more out of it.

They may find they aren't exhausted anymore too because life has slowed down for them. They may be retired now so the daily grind of work isn't causing them to go to bed so tired they can't even think about sex. They have plenty of time to spend looking and feeling good. This means they can also spend more time with their partner.

As many individuals know, having a quality relationship on other levels with your partner leads to better sex. You may find that now that you have time to spend with each other on fun activities instead of just household chores you enjoy each other more. It can bring an entirely new level of intimacy to the bedroom for you as well.

Many people over 60 that are retired also travel. The excitement of seeing new places with someone you have a sexual relationship with can rejuvenate your sex drive as well. You may find new locations for the activity to take place is quite a turn on. Where you are and what activities you are enjoying can also play a role in that.

Not everyone will have such an increase in their sexual behavior though as they get older. Some people may really want to have sex more often but their body isn't cooperating. They may find it harder to get or maintain an erection for the act to take place. This can lead to a great deal of embarrassment as well as anxiety.

The body may just simply start to feel older and more worn down too. This can result in a person having less sexual activity than they did before. It can be frustrating when a person isn't ready for these issues to take place. Sometimes you can get results if you take to a doctor. Other times you will have to be able to come to terms with some changes in your sexual behavior that are the result of aging.

Talking to a counselor about it can be very helpful as well. Some older individuals become depressed when they find their sexual relationship isn't what it once was. They may blame themselves for it and need help to cope. Others may become angry at their spouse due to their changed feelings towards sexual activity. It is very important for the relationship to be open enough to discuss such matters.

Dealing with changes in your sexual relationship when you are 60 or older may not be your cup of tea, but you may find you have no choice. You may be pleasantly surprised to find that sex gets better for you as you get older. You may also find that the best is behind you. Yet you can still have a good time with it if you are willing to make some adjustments.

5- Tips for Adults over 60 with Heart Disease to still Enjoy Sex

Heart disease is one of the biggest killers of both men and women in our society. It is very important to take care of it. One fear that many people over the age of 60 have is that their heart disease will put a damper on their sex life. There are ways to effectively control your heart disease though and still be able to enjoy a very active and fulfilling sex life.

Heart disease can result in a person having to take medications for the duration of their life. Many of these medications have proven to be successful but not without a cost. There can be various side effects with them such as erectile dysfunction. This means a male can't maintain an erection. Most doctors won't prescribe various types of medication to help with it such as Viagra or Cialis though if you don't have a healthy enough heart to be engaging in sex in the first place.

Of course there is the common fear in our society that anyone who has heart disease could die due to the excitement of sex. There have been reports of heart attacks and other issues occurring during sex for those with heart disease. While these instances do occur, they are often very few and far between. Still, if your doctor tells you to change your habits and that you can't engage in various types of sexual activities you need to listen.

In most instances though your sex life doesn't have to come to a screeching halt. Instead you may find there are some modifications to be made. You need to be open to the suggestions and the changes though as they may prove to be more satisfying to you than you thought. Remember that your overall health is very crucial and so you need to be disciplined about sticking to the set boundaries by your health car professionals.

Make sure you are following all of the orders like you should. This means taking daily medications on time. Eat meals that are healthy for you so that you can keep up your energy. Pay attention to signs from your body that something just isn't right. If you get dizzy or short of breath during sexual activities then you may need to stop what you are doing.

Having a loving and caring partner though all of this is extremely important. That can help to reduce your level of stress and anxiety. They should be willing to forego various types of sexual activity in order to help you stay as healthy as possible. You may find that making various changes to your lifestyle though helps. You may be able to resume old forms of lovemaking in the future if you are willing to stick to such necessary changes.

Heart disease is a very serious issue and you should do all you can at a young age to prevent it from occurring. You want to be as healthy as you can when you get into your 60's and beyond. It will ensure you have a happier lifestyle that also includes being able to enjoy various types of sexual activities.

Should you end up with heart disease though due to poor lifestyle choices or due to heredity, you can still find ways to enjoy sex. It is important to discuss the issue with your doctor though. You certainly don't want to be engaging in any types of behavior that aren't in your best interest.

6- The Internet is the Perfect Place for those over 60 to Freely Discuss Sex

The generation gap is alive and well when it comes to many issues in our society. Sex is one of them and so the older generations are turning to the internet as the perfect place to feely talk about it. There younger co-workers, friends, and certainly their own children don't want to discuss it with them. It can be hard for younger generations to accept the fact the their own parents and even grandparents are still having sex.

Yet more and more people are living a healthier lifestyle to late in life. This means there is no reason why someone over the age of 60 can't be having the time of their life when it comes to their sexual relationships. It doesn't matter if they have been with the same person for years or if they are newly on the market and seeing what it has to offer them.

Not everyone from the older generations is comfortable talking openly about sex. They may feel guilty or embarrassed about doing so. Yet with the internet you can talk freely to others and hide behind the screen. No one ever has to find out your real name or what you look like. You may be talking online with people in another country or just across town from you. The anonymous nature of the internet though makes it safe and so people tend to open up more.

There is a great deal of information to be found online too about how sex is for those over 60. Individuals who are experiencing low libido or a variety of other problems that are sexual in nature can find out more about it. They can get support because they know that they aren't alone in what they are going though.

In many instances, reading such information can help them come to terms with where they are. They may be encouraged to go see a doctor or a counselor to help them get passed the issue. They may find that they are able to rid themselves of the guilt associated with having sex with a new partner after their previous one died. All of these issues and more are covered in great detail online for those that are 60 and older.

A person can simply choose to read articles that are posted online. Search engines are a great way to be able to narrow down the topics. As you read more articles you can jot down notes. This way you can come up with more keywords to enter and do other searches on. You can collect the information you want from the privacy of your home without feeling self conscious about it.

There are also plenty of forums where other people can read your posts and respond to them. This is a great way to get personalize information that is specific to the questions you have. You can also do your part by reading what others need and responding. This is a great way to give back the support that has been given to you along your road to sexual happiness at an older age.

It seems that there are more and more individuals older than 60 out there sharing their stories of having sex. Some of them are fun while others are full of questions. You do need to make sure that you get reliable information though. Just because there is something written on the internet doesn't make it true. Take the time to verify the resources. Keep in mind that a great deal of the information you do come across will be the personal opinions of other adults and not based on anything credible by and expert.

Still, what you do get from other people who have been through similar experiences can give you something to think about. It can help you to overcome personal fears as well as provide you with some comical relief from time to time.

7- Ways for Men over 60 to Deal with Erectile Dysfunction

As a man gets older the ability to get and to maintain an erection can be harder. Some men find it just takes a bit more foreplay. They may also find they can't get a second erection soon after like they once could. This is normal and most couples find it to be an issue they can easily deal with. They are still able to have a very satisfying sex life in spite of such minor issues.

However, some males end up with what is know as erectile dysfunction. This can become a serious issue that affects the individual both mentally and physically. At first they may only have the problem once in a while. It can be embarrassing but couples can deal with it. The partner needs to be very encouraging and supportive so it won't become a mental issue the next time sex is initiated.

For other men though erectile dysfunction can end up being a very serious problem. It can result in them becoming angry or upset. It can also lead to depression as many men do associate their manhood with their ability to have sexual intercourse. There are many reasons why a man may suffer from erectile dysfunction when they are 60 or older.

Medical concerns are the number one factor. Heart disease, high blood pressure, and even diabetes can all cause erectile dysfunction. Seeing a professional about what is going on is very important. They can help prescribe medications that can help with the issue. Sometimes it turns out to be the medications that you are on that make it hard to get an erection. The doctor can help to determine the cause and get the person back on track.

Mentally a man can prevent himself from being able to get an erection. Issues about not being able to in the past can certainly cause a great deal of anxiety. Not feeling attractive or worrying about being able to perform can also be a problem. Talking to your partner about your fears can help to alleviate them.

Changing lifestyle habits can really make a difference too. Some men over 60 aren't able to get an erection due to heavily smoking or drinking. Working to get rid of these habits can help the issue of erectile dysfunction to take care of itself. Likewise, changing your diet and losing weight can be helpful as well.

There are several reasons why males over 60 years of age may be experiencing erectile dysfunction. Yet it doesn't have to mean the very end of your sexual lifestyle. There are ways to deal with it that can get you back on track again. Be willing to try different things in order to get to the bottom of your problem.

One of the most frustrating things for men with erectile dysfunction is that it can take time to discover what is going to make a difference. You have to be willing to follow the doctor's orders. You have to be open to trying a course of action for a couple of months and then exploring another one if that one wasn't effective for you.

Sex for men over 60 is still very important and it can be very fulfilling. Don't be afraid to look at your lifestyle to see where you can make changes. Go to a doctor you can trust and you are comfortable with. This way you can share your feelings and discover what your options are for effectively dealing with erectile dysfunction.

Some of the different treatments that a doctor can offer include various medications. With advances in technology there are also implants that are surgically placed inside of the penis. Counseling can be very effective when the doctor feels there may be a mental link to the erectile dysfunction. Exploring the various options can help you to be able to get and maintain an erection again like you did when you were younger.

8- Safe Sex is Still a Concern for those Over 60 Years of Age

Just because you get older, it doesn't mean you can be careless about your choice of sexual partners. For those over 60 years of age, you want to do your part to protect yourself. Both men and women need to take the responsibility for having condoms readily available. While they risk of pregnancy is likely in the past, the risk of sexually transmitted diseases is not.

Most individuals over the age of 60 aren't out hooking up with new partners every weekend. Yet the biggest concern should be the people they have been with in the past. They may have been exposed to a sexually transmitted diseases such as HIV from a partner they were once with. They aren't able to share that information with you as they don't know it themselves. That is just too big of a risk to take.

Should you decide to be part of a committed relationship when you are over 60 with one partner, that is great. You both should be tested for sexually transmitted diseases though. The time frame for additional testing will depend on how much time has passed since each of you has been with someone else. Your medical professionals can provide all of that information for you.

Only after you get go ahead for the doctor can you stop using protection with that partner. You need to decide on the level of trust you have with that person though. Infidelity is a common issue in our society for people of all ages, not just over 60. If you are worried in the least that you may be exposed to anything due to that issue you need to continue using protection.

It is very naïve to assume that because you aren't a spring chicken anymore that you don't have to worry about the risk of sexually transmitted diseases. There is no discrimination from them based upon your age. Approximately 20% of the population that has tested positive for HIV is over 60 years of age. In at least half of the cases it is believed that they were exposed to the virus by engaging in unprotected sex after the age of 60.

Some individuals of this age group feel it is disrespectful to bring up the use of condoms. They don't want to offend potential partners so they don't even bring it up. Yet if you aren't able to discuss the issue of safe sex with someone you plan to be intimate with then it is best to avoid such activity with them all together.

Others simply don't realize they are still at risk at their age. There has been a great deal of information and education offered on the topic in the last 20 years. This was implemented as the number of individuals over 60 years of age with sexually transmitted diseases was on the rise for several years in a row.

The highest rate of sexually transmitted diseases among adults of this age group is found in male to male relationships. However, those that involve two females or one male and one female are also at risk too. There has been a myth in society that doesn't seem to go away that only homosexual males are at risk of contracting a sexually transmitted disease in their older years. Everyone is at risk and so you should assume that anyone you are going to have sex with could possible have such infections to pass on to you. Some of them may know about it but others don't and you need to not take such a risk.

When you are in your 60's, you still have plenty of life ahead of you to enjoy. A healthy sex life should be a an enjoyable part of that life. However, you do need to be very realistic about the risk of sexually transmitted diseases. You don't want to have something like that affect the quality of the remainder of life you have in front of you

9- When you are Older than 60 and Sex is no Longer an Interest to you

Don't assume that just because you will one day be 60 years of age that sex won't interest you. There isn't going to be a day when you wake up and say that is the last time you will be engaging in such events. There is plenty of talk about those over 60 that pursue an active and healthy sex life. Yet not everyone falls into that category. There are some that are just no longer interested in it.

You do owe it to yourself though to find out why you aren't interested in having sex. For many it has to do with the loss of a partner due to death. They may have been with that individual for a very long time. They simply can't imagine themselves becoming intimate with anyone else. This is understandable and not something that should be viewed as out of the ordinary.

There is no set time frame for a person to recover from such events. Eventually you may feel like you are ready to see someone new. It may be within the year or several years down the road. Listen to your own feelings and follow your heart. If you are struggling to let go of the past, professional counseling may be something you can benefit from.

There are those who never really enjoyed sex in the first place. They continued to do it because they felt it was expected from them. They may have wanted to have children or just to keep the peace with their spouse. They may be at a point in their life where they just don't feel that sex is that important anymore. They also aren't going to compromise their stand on it for anyone else any longer.

Some individuals are very concerned about their physical appearance. They go to great lengths as they get older to look their very best. They chose their clothing very carefully so they can accent their good qualities and hide their flaws. So they aren't about to show someone what they look like naked.

Medical issues are one of the main reasons why some people over the age of 60 just don't find sex to be of interest. They may be very ill and it is a fight daily to go about their normal activities. Others find they have a very low libido due to their medical problems or even as a side effect of their medications. Therefore the issue of sex just isn't one that matters a great deal to them.

Likewise, if they have a partner who is suffering from various medical problems they may find that sex doesn't matter. They are more concerned with helping their partner to remain as comfortable as they possibly can. It takes tremendous strength to help someone with daily medical problems. It can be physically and mentally draining as well. Yet at the end of the day they are just thankful to continue having more time to share with that person.

When you are older than 60 and sex is no longer an interest to you, that is your own concern. You need to make sure you are truly happy with that decision though. If you find you are depressed about it or long for some type of sexual activity you need to see a doctor. There can be many reasons why a person isn't able to enjoy sex as they get older. There are numerous solutions that can be offered as well. If you aren't interested in them though you can still have wonderful and meaningful relationships.

You will just have to find a partner who isn't interested in sex either. Otherwise that different between the two of you is going to end up creating a great deal of tension. As long as both of you are fine with only being companions then it can work well for you. Sex isn't something anyone should feel pressured into at any age.

10- Natural Ways to Rejuvenate your Sex Life for those Older than 60

If you want to have a better sex life later in life then you do now, you can work to rejuvenate it. When was the last time you really took some time to pamper yourself? If it has been a while then take some time to do so. Go get a new outfit and a hair cut or color. Buy some new make up and plan a romantic dinner for you and your partner.

Allow yourself some time to fantasize about sex during the day as well. Take a nice warm bath before bed. You can picture what you will do with your partner when you are done with the bath. Leave them a detailed note in the morning about plans for the evening. It can certainly make a huge difference in the way you see each other romantically. Keep it fresh and alive so that no one gets bored with the sexual activity that is taking place.

Take a look at your mental well being as well. If you aren't in the best of moods then do what you can to perk yourself up. Sometimes seeing a professional counselor can help you out as well. Sometimes there are issues not dealt with in the relationship that lead to tension and resentment. If you can get them on the table and out of the way your sex life will likely improve.

Taking care of yourself physically is important as well. Don't let yourself get lazy or overweight. Stay active and eat well so you can stay at a healthy weight. You may need to work with a dietician to plan healthier meals. It is never too late in life to make such lifestyle changes. It does take some planning and commitment but your will find there are many great benefits from it.

Get rid of those nasty habits such as excessively drinking alcohol. In the long run it will lower your sexual desire and performance, especially for men. Smoking is also a factor that will become more of an issue as you get older. Being comfortable in your own skin and with how you look is a great way to get you in the mood to initiate sexual activity with your partner as well. They will find it to be a tremendous turn on that you are attracted to them.

Sometimes just changing the location of where sex will take place can make it better. If you are always doing the act at home, take a weekend vacation to some place romantic. You can also use a different room in the house to spice it up a bit. There are books on new positions and even on romancing your partner to look at as well. You may find talking honestly with your partner about how to please them can really make a difference.

There are herbal pills for both men and women on the market as well. Since you can buy them over the counter at most health food stores people assume they are 100% safe to take. Still, you need to consult with your doctor first. You may not be healthy enough to engage in sexual activity. You certainly don't want to risk your health for sex so getting a full assessment from a professional is the best place to start.

11- How Happy are those in their 60's with their Sex Life?

It may surprise you to find out how happy many people in their 60's are with their sex life. This is due to people living longer lives than ever before due to effective health care. We also know how important it is to take care of our bodies. Sex isn't something that has to go out the window just because you have aged. In fact, more people that are 60 years of age or older are having a great time with it than you might think.

The act of those over 60 enjoying sex isn't something new though like many people think. What has changed though is that there is more freedom to talk about it and to express information about it. You can even find places online where these people are talking about their sexual feelings and experiences. There are also many people in this age group still dating.

Since they are on the dating scene, it is reasonable to expect that they will one day take those relationships to another level. They can have a very satisfying sexual lifestyle that helps keep them both young and vibrant. In fact, there is information to suggest that the more sexually active individuals are as they get older the happier they will be.

Not everyone in this age group is happy with their sex life though. Women tend to have more problems with it then men. This is because there are more women in those older age groups than men. Not all of them are comfortable being with younger men due to how they feel society is going to see it. Yet there is really nothing wrong with it if both parties are happy with the relationship.

For males, the inability to maintain an erection is the number one reason why they aren't happy with their sex life in their 60's. Yet there are many ways in which this problem can be resolved. Most doctors can help men get to the core of the issue and then let them know what options they have. Just because a person is older and things aren't working on their own like they one did doesn't mean you have to let it continue to be that way.

Being sexually intimate is a great way to for older individuals to feel that they are loved and appreciated. They certainly don't want to be lonely as they get older. Even if they do have friends and family, nothing can make you feel as wonderful as the respect and admiration from someone else. It is a good feeling to know someone desires you sexually as well.

Don't under estimate the power of having a sex life you are happy with at any age. It can only become more rewarding as an individual gets older. If you are over 60 and not happy with your sex life, then you do have the power to change it. Take an honest look at what you are happy with and what you aren't.

Once you have done this, evaluate what can be done to change it. These factors will fall into one of three categories – what you can do on your own, what you can do with your partner, and what you can change with the help of your doctor. Those things you can change on your own include your attitude towards sex, your feelings towards your body, and getting into touch with your feelings.

You can make sex more rewarding when you are older by asking your partner to tell you what they need to make it more pleasurable. At the same time, express what the do that turns you on and what you need more of. If you find you don't enjoy sex like you used to then you should speak to your doctor about what can be done.

12- Will you Still have an Active Sex Life in your 60's?

Sex is a very important part of life for most people, and very natural as well. It seems that it is more of a big deal for younger individuals than those who are older. Maybe it is because they have learned what a relationship is all about by then, and sex is just a small portion of it. Still, it is important and something that you will want to still be a part of.

One of the biggest problems though is that people aren't comfortable with their bodies as they get older. It is true that things may not be where they used to be, and wrinkles may be in place. Yet if you are able to love your body for what it is, sex in your 60's can still be very enjoyable.

Some individuals around this age have been with the same partner for decades. They are very comfortable with them. They are still able to have a satisfying sexual relationship because they know what their partner finds enjoyable. It is never too late to start experimenting either!

Others around this age group are with a new partner for a variety of reasons. They may have been divorced and focused on their career or children. Now they are ready to focus on their own personal happiness. A new love interest in your 60's can be very exciting for someone. It can be something for you to appreciate if companionship and love is something you are looking for in your life.

Part of being able to enjoy an active sex life in your 60's has to do with your health as well. It is important to have regular check ups so that your doctor can assess any problems you may be experiencing. You also need to stay active because that going to increase your level of energy and endurance for sexual activities.

You may find you have more time to exercise on a regular basis at this time in your life. You likely don't have children to care for at home and you may be very close to retirement. There are plenty of walking clubs and exercise groups for older individuals where you can make some great friends too. This may help you to look forward to exercising when you saw it as a burden before.

Not everyone finds that sex is that important when they are in their 60's though. It is important for you and your partner to be able to communicate what your sexual needs and interests are. If you are both content with it only happening once in a while that is fine. If you both would like it to take place regularly then that is fine too.

Should you discover that your sexual needs and desires are very different from each other though it could pose problems for your relationship. If you are open and honest about your needs and feelings though you can find it to be something you can work out as a couple. Both individuals should be looking forward to the sexual activity rather than one feeling pressured into participating.

Sex can be a wonderful experience at any age. If you enjoy it and you are healthy enough for it, there is no reason why you can't continue it into your 60's and beyond. If you find you don't enjoy it as much as you once did, there may be some things you can do about that. Talk to your doctor and you can come up with some solutions together.

13- Having Sex into your 60's and Beyond can help you Feel Younger

When we are young we often proudly tell people just how old we are. That all changes though when a person gets older. However, you are only truly as old as you feel. Skip the skin cream if you want to feel younger as one of the best ways to do so is to have a good sex life. Some will argue that this isn't always possible due to not having a partner, but even masturbating when you are 60 or older will help you to feel younger.

Sexual activity helps to relieve tension in both the mind and the body. It is agreed that all adults can certainly benefit from that. A healthy sex life also helps you to feel good about who you are. There are few things in life that are as intimate between two individuals as having sexual relations. If you are true to the meaning behind your feelings then sex can only get better for you as you get older.

It may be hard for younger generations to understand how sex can get better with age. It has to do with the emotional connection that is found in the older years. We often take our relationships for granted when we are younger even if we truly do love those we are with. The physical as well as the emotional connect that can be made is what makes it that much more special.

You can feel younger having sex when you are past your 60th birthday and have some additional perks. For example you often don't have to worry about work schedules, taking care of children, or many other types of interruptions that can get into your way. There is also no longer a risk of getting pregnant and that can allow many couples to feel very free.

When you are young, you often can't imagine being over 60 and still having sex. It may seem like you are going to be so old. It really depends on your age when you start having such thoughts though. Keep in mind that your physical condition is going to affect how old you feel. Some 40 year olds physically feel older than many 60 years old. Staying active is going to be key to being able to still enjoy sex at an older age.

You may not have experimented much with sex when you were younger but still have the desire to do so. You are never too old to have fun with sex so let your partner know what your desires are. Chances are they will be very willing to comply with what you want to be fulfilled. Make sure you find out what they need as well so both of you can enjoy the activities and feel younger in the process.

Sex is an activity that people can really enjoy for their entire adult life. It doesn't have to stop just because of the number of candles on your birthday cake. While it is true that you won't hear as many 60 something people talking about sex, they are still enjoying it. There are plenty of statistics out there that reflect this. You can feel good about yourself as well as feel years younger if you are actively enjoying sex at this age and beyond.

14- Maintaining your Sex Drive as you get Older

Maintaining your sex drive as you get older is very important to most people. Sex is a satisfying part of their lifestyle and not one they want to lose. It is normal for a person's sex drive to diminish some though as they get older. Specifically those over 60 may find it is harder to get into the mood or even to get your body to physically comply with what you want to do.

There are some things you can do though to help you maintain your sex drive as you get older. Living a healthy lifestyle is going to make a very significant impact for you so don't blow it off. What you choose to do today is going to affect your health and your level of sexual desire as you get older.

Eating a well balanced diet is something you should incorporate into your life. If you aren't doing it now, then start to make some small changes. As time goes on you will adjust to them and they will become a second nature to you. Consuming too much caffeine can be a problem. If you aren't getting all the vitamins and nutrients that you need from food, make sure you take a quality supplement.

Make sure you take the time to exercise at least 30 minutes each day as well. Walking is very common for older individuals as it is low impact but very good for the body. Get a companion such as a friend or even a dog that you can walk with each day. Some malls and other locations have indoor walking clubs too which are perfect when the weather turns cold.

Maintaining a healthy weight is very important to sex drive. A combination of a good diet with plenty of exercise will help you to be successful in this area. It will also help you to feel great about how you look. Too many people are inhibited about sex as their body has changed from what it once was. That is going to be a fact of life for all of us.

Being happy with your body is also important. Too many people start to notice all the small details as they get older. They will see every line and wrinkle on their body so they aren't comfortable during sex. They don't have much self confidence that they are desirable. They aren't able to let go and enjoy what is taking place because they are too focused on such details.

Reducing the amount of stress in your life is important as you get older too. The toll it can take on both your body and your mind is more than most of us imagine. Not everyone can be worry free when they are older though. If your finances or relationships aren't in the best format, it can be hard to get past it. Do your very best though to reduce as many stressful issues from your life as you can. It will certainly help with your sex drive because you won't be preoccupied with other things.

If you are healthy as you get older, you will be able to maintain your sex drive. Both men and women have the ability to be turned on sexually until a very late age in life. They also both have the ability to continue having orgasms into those later years as well. It all comes down to how fit a person is though both physically and mentally.

Age is merely a number though as anyone who is over 60 can tell you. Many of them continue to enjoy as wonderful of a sex life as others who are only in their 40's. It is something you can strive for in your own life as well. Make sure you are making healthy choices today though so you won't have too many issues that reduce your sex drive as you get older.

15- Statistics Regarding Sexual Activity for those Over 60

You may be surprised by the statistics for those over 60 enjoying sex. Women aren't just sitting at home knitting while their men are out on the golf course. Instead they are enjoying each other physically and that is good news. More than half of all individuals who are at least 60 years of age are engaging in sexual intercourse.

You may be curious about how often this is taking place. 22% say that they engage in sexual activity at least one a week. 28% of them say that they engage in sexual activity at least one a month. When you consider how many people in our society fall into that age group then we have something great to look forward to.

Even with more than half of all people over 60 engaging in sexual activity, approximately 39% will tell you they want more. It could be that they aren't involved in a relationship right now that is going anywhere. Others may be looking for the right person to be intimate with but it just hasn't happened yet. You will find casual sexual encounters among those over 60 don't often happen as they do for those in their 20's and 30's.

Almost 95% of adults over 60 will admit in surveys to participating in the act of masturbating. Many believe this is something that older people don't do. Yet that isn't the truth of the matter at all. More males engage in masturbating over the age of 60 than women though. Many men say it helps them to be able to stay healthy and to get an erection when they do want to have sex with their partner.

However, approximately 75% of those that fit into this category will tell you that they are enjoying the sex they are having. They feel aroused, they feel desired, and they definitely are benefiting from the activity. Both men and women continue to be able to achieve an orgasm at this age. It may take longer to become aroused but the end result doesn't seem to have changed.

Almost all women who are over 60 will tell you that sex today is better than it was for them twenty years ago. Many of them are still with the same partner. They just find that they have more freedom in their life now when it comes to sex. They also have learned to better communicate to their partner what it takes to arouse and satisfy them.

Men are five times more likely than women to not be able to perform sexually due to medical problems. Heart disease is a problem that can affect both men and women in this age group. Yet men can also suffer from erectile dysfunction due to their various medical problems.

Both men and women in this age group may find that they don't seem to feel as attractive as they once did. 16% of them will tell you they don't have sex as often as they would like to because of it. They may wait until the conditions are right such as it being completely dark.

The statistics regarding sexual activity for those over 60 can be viewed as quite accurate. These days more people that fall into that age group are proud of their sexual activities. They are very willing to share that information with others who ask. They also take parent in online surveys where they can share opinions but still maintain their anonymity.

Based on this information, those getting older shouldn't be too worried about their sexual lifestyle. In fact, many people over 60 will tell you that they have a better sex life now than they did just 10 years ago. It may be due to how they now feel about their body or just a change in their routine. Regardless, sex over 60 is definitely something you can look forward to.

16- How Menopause can Decrease Sexual Desire for Women over 60

There are some significant changes that take place in a woman's life. One of them is menopause. This marks the end of her ability to conceive a child. There will be no more menstrual cycles once the woman is in complete menopause. Yet it can take years to go from the start of menopause to completely finishing it. Most women start the process around 45 and finish around 60. It can be sooner or later though as each woman is different.

There is a common misconception that women who have gone through menopause no longer have any sexual desire. They may continue to engage in the activity to keep their partner happy, but they don't get any pleasure out of it. This is certainly not the truth though.

Many women over the age of 60 are involved in very fulfilling sexual relationships. They love not having to worry about their period. They also don't have to worry about an unwanted pregnancy very late in life. This new found freedom for them means they are able to fully focus on the act of sexual activity and not the various repercussions of it.

Some women do experience a drop in their sexual desire though after menopause. Many women experience problems with the vagina being dry after menopause. This can make it hard for them to get pleasure out of sexual activity. There are some great products on the market though that will allow you to moisturize the vagina without any negative side effects.

It is a good idea for a woman with such issues to see a gynecologist for a complete evaluation though. They may be able to help come up with a natural remedy that can prevent ongoing issues having to be addressed with it. For many women, dealing with vaginal dryness can cause a mental block with sexual intercourse.

They may connect it with being undesirable now that they are in their 60's. This low self confidence can cause women to shy away from sexual intercourse as well. Being able to really enjoy your body and your sexual desires when you are over 60 is very important. It will encourage you to do what you can to be able to bring back a high level of sexual desire to your life.

Sometimes something over the counter though isn't enough for a woman to get back the sexual desire she once had. Your doctor may offer you supplements of hormones in the form of estrogen. Since the level of it in the body drops dramatically due to menopause, replacing it definitely can be helpful.

Menopause doesn't have to hinder your sex life though for women over 60 years of age. If you enjoy sex and you want to continue doing so, there are remedies out there that can help. Don't be embarrassed to discuss the issue with your doctor either. They deal with such issues all the time. They will know how to help you get back to where you want to be sexually.

For many older couples, menopause can throw a wrench into what was once a very enjoyable part of their intimate relationship. It is important to discuss what has taken place. A woman doesn't want her partner to assume the lack of sexual responsiveness has anything to do with them not being attractive anymore. Find a good solution that works for you so that menopause won't stop you from engaging your sexual relationship.

17- Common Causes of Erectile Dysfunction for Males Older than 60

Erectile dysfunction can definitely hurt a man's physical and mental ability to enjoy sex. Even if he is turned on by a woman and wants to complete the act, the body simply isn't going to comply. This is an event that just about every single man out there will experience at least once in their life, especially as they get older. It isn't a big deal unless it is happening on a regular basis.

The key to getting past it though is to realize that you aren't alone. Too many men hide their issue with erectile dysfunction from everyone. They are too embarrassed to tell their partner so they may look for reasons to avoid sexual activity. They can pick fights, become distant, and even make the partner feel bad about their appearance to cast blame in another direction.

For those not in a serious relationship, erectile dysfunction can prevent it from occurring. They know that eventually a new relationship will get to the point where sex should be taking place They don't want any women to find out they can't perform so they withdraw from women in a social setting all together.

It is important for men to realize that there are many common causes for erectile dysfunction. Therefore there is no reason to feel inadequate about the process taking place. It is going to be a natural part of getting older for many men. A doctor can often help to identify what the cause of the problem is though and help a man get his sex life back.

Vascular disease accounts for more than half of all the erectile dysfunction cases in males over the age of 60. This has to do with the arteries to the penis getting blocked and so not enough blood can get to it for a full erection. This is a condition that can often be treated though.

Smoking is a common issue that can lead to it as well. Males who smoke more than a pack of cigarettes per day are at the highest risk. Stopping to smoke can make a huge difference for the individual in just a month or two.

There are a variety of medical problems that can lead to erectile dysfunction for men. The biggest one though is diabetes. The nerved and blood vessels to the penis may be damaged and so there isn't enough blood that is allowed to flow into it for an erection to take place.

When we hear about hormone problems and sexual behavior for those over 60, it is mostly associated with women. Yet approximately 5% of all males suffer from some type of hormone problem. That is what is responsible for their problems with getting an erection. They may have a problem with their kidneys or liver due to hereditary illnesses or excessive alcohol use.

Some men fail to product enough testosterone as they get older so they need a supplement to help with their sex drive. There are also times when traumatic experiences can affect the normal ability to get an erection. It could be due to an injury that harms the spine or even due to the onset of various diseases that affect the central nervous system.

Doctors have to be careful about prescribing medications for various ailments as well. All prescription drugs have side effects and hundreds of them have impotency as one of them. Since many of these drugs have to be taken on a daily basis it is a huge concern. These various medications may be to treat heart disease, diabetes, depression, or anxiety. It is important for a doctor to try to find a good medication that works but doesn't affect the ability to obtain and maintain a natural erection.

With all the technology available today, that is no reason for a man over 60 to suffer from no sex life. There are simply too many ways in which they can be helped. However, this help can't be offered unless they are open and willing to discuss their sexual problems with professionals.

18- Why do So Many Women Enjoy Sex more when they are over 60?

There is often a belief in society that men enjoy sex much more than women. For many years overall this is true. Women often worry about issues such as pregnancy, they have their hands full with too many things, or they aren't happy with their body. Yet they continue to engage in sexual activities as a way to keep their partner happy. Women are very good at doing what is going to keep others happy. It is often a part of their very giving nature.

Some women continue to engage in sex during their life as they want to be able to enjoy it more. They may experiment with new methods as well as new partners. All the while though it may just be something they go through the motions of. Women often associate the act of sex with intimacy afterwards so they do it in order to get to that part of it.

It is often said that many women enjoy sex more as they get older. There are many researchers who will tell you it has to do with changes in the body. A woman may find it easier to have an orgasm when she is in her 30's. She may have come to terms with how her body looks or be with the same partner long enough to be very comfortable communicating what it is that she wants.

This results in sex becoming something that a woman can enjoy and look forward to when she is older. It has more to do with intimacy than with just being sexy for someone. Since sex isn't the core of the relationship when you are older than 60, the pressure is off a woman to look perfect and to perform perfectly. This can help it to be something enjoyable instead of another time when she continues to critic herself.

There is said to be a great deal of passion in the sexual aspect of things for older couples. This is because it focuses more on the feelings involved than just the act itself. The woman finds her partner is taking more time for touching and caressing which is exactly what women crave when it comes to sex.

All of this pampering and personal attention for women past 60 years of age may be something new. They may not have had such experiences with sex when they were younger. While most men won't admit it, they often focused on their own sexual needs when they were younger as well. Older men are known to be able to please a woman better.

More women are opening up to tell others how much they enjoy sex into their 60's and older. This used to be a taboo subject so it was just assumed that they didn't really participate in it or enjoy it. Yet that seems to be very far from the truth. Researchers have found that women will open up about their sexual activities when they are older if someone is directly asking the questions.

There are many reasons why women find sex after 60 to be extremely gratifying. They are able to continue to enjoy this part of their life regardless of their age. It is exciting to have the freedom to explore their sexuality. They also love the fact that their partner finds them interesting and wants to have sex with them. This can really help a person who is getting older to feel very good about themselves.

19- Health Issues for Men that can Make Sex over 60 Difficult

By the time a man is 60 years of age, his normal level of sexual intercourse has dropped by half. This is based on the average peak from around 18 to 25 years of age for a normal male. There are a variety of different health issues for men that can make engaging in sex after they are 60 years of age difficult.

There are both physical and mental problems for men that can make it difficult to get or maintain an erection. Even if the problems starts out being physical in nature, it can soon turn into a psychological issue as well. This is because a man can feel inadequate when he can no longer fulfill this role. He may become angry, upset, and even emotionally withdrawn because of it.

Even during sexual excitement, he may be thinking about it in the back of his mind. The anxiety of previously not being able to get or maintain an erection can certainly affect a man. The fear of it happening again can actually cause it to happen to the point where a man will avoid engaging in any type of intimacy that could lead to the woman wanting sexual intercourse to take place.

A male may find that various medications that have to be taken for medical problems can result in erectile dysfunction. The is can be frustrating because in order to take care of a certain medical need they have to give up something that is giving them a great deal of pleasure. Taking the medication may only be temporary but if it is to be an ongoing need then it is more of a concern.

Sometimes the erectile dysfunction from the medications is a side effect that goes away as the body adjusts to it. Other times the doctor is going to need to adjust the dosage or even try out new medications. Many males don't want to share this problem with their doctor though so they just stop taking their medication. That is certainly not a good solution for any male who is having problems with sex due to medication conditions as well as their age.

There are some healthy issues for men that make sex after the age of 60 difficult that are more on the mental level than anything else. They may find they don't have the same defined look in their arms or abs that they once had. They may find it hard to believe a woman still wants to be with them sexually when they look like that.

Low self esteem is a major problem for men with their overall physical appearance as they get older. The development of a beer gut or even the onset of going bald can all affect them. Do your best to remind yourself of your best qualities so you can focus on having a great time during sex and not your appearance.

Not all males over the age of 60 will have health issues that prevent them from having a happy sex life. However, since so many well it is a very important issue to address. They can become frustrated when they can no longer perform sexually as they once did. It can create issues in their relationship too if their partner no longer feels desired or their sexual needs aren't being satisfied.

20- Vascular Disease can Create Complications for Men over 60 wishing to have Sex

Vascular disease is a type of problem older males can experience. It is a type of erectile dysfunction so it can definitely affect their ability to have the quality of sexual lifestyle they are interested in. With vascular disease, the arteries end up hardening. This is going to prevent enough blood from being able to flow to the penis for it to get hard at all or to get hard enough for intercourse to take place.

Approximately 60% of all men over the age of 60 who have a type of erectile dysfunction find that it is due to vascular disease. This is why men over the age of 55 are encouraged to get a screening annually. Most doctors will include it in the physical exam that they do. Yet too many males don't see a doctor for a routine check up each year as they should. As a result, they end up with vascular disease being a problem that isn't identified until it has already affected their ability to maintain an erection.

The research on the cases of vascular disease that have been found find some common factors. Males who smoke, have high cholesterol, or that are overweight tend to be at a higher risk. Males who have been diagnosed with diabetes or heart disease also have a higher chance of developing vascular disease as well.

In order to determine if a man is suffering from vascular disease, an assessment is completed. Generally a blood test is done which can provide the necessary information. The penis may be touched as well to determine how sensitive the nerves are in it in connection with arousal.

It is also very important for the patient to give accurate information. The assessment will ask when they last time a full erection was maintained. Many men lie about it as they don't want to face the problem or share it with their doctor. Yet they are there to help with such issues and not being honest can prevent you from having a great sex life.

Once the vascular disease has been confirmed, the doctor can discuss the course or action to remedy it. Many men who need to make lifestyle changes such as to stop smoking or to lose weight will for sexual activity to take place. That is how important it is to them and the life they wish to engage in.

Sometimes the physical issues of vascular disease have to be treated with emotional needs too. For the male who has been dealing with it for a while, the anxiety and shame of not being able to maintain an erection can be a factor. Even if the physical issues are resolved, the mental block is still going to be there. Dealing with both factors at once gives these men the best chance of overcoming their erectile dysfunction.

Depending on the assessment, the man may be given a prescription for various types of medications to help maintain an erection. Many of them have been quite successful and they continue to improve all the time. There are also vacuum devices given that will help to pull more blood into the penis so the erection can take place.

Surgery is becoming more of a common way to treat vascular disease that has lead to erectile dysfunction as well. Many men want to go this route rather than having to use drugs or a pump to get their erections to take place. With surgery the arteries can be cleared so that the blood can naturally flow to the penis like it should. If there are veins that allow the blood to leak out they can be blocked. There are also implants that can be permanently inserted to assist a man with getting an erection.

An estimated 30 million men are affected by vascular disease right now. Finding out if you are at risk is important as it can help you to avoid being part of the statistics. Should you end up with vascular disease though there are very effective ways of treating it. Rather than giving up on sex, see a doctor who can help you find the right solution for you.

21- Some Common Problems for Women Older than 60 that can Make Sex Uncomfortable

Sex can continue for women at any age, but there are some common problems that can affect those over 60 and make it uncomfortable. If you aren't feeling good during the activity of course it is going to be something you avoid being a part of. That can really make you feel less attractive and even older than you really are. Sex is a big part of who we are even though it isn't the most important attribute.

Too many women just sum up these common problems as the end of a very happy sex life. Others never really enjoyed it anyway so now it is just one more issue to prevent them from considering sex as something wonderful or rewarding. Yet you don't have to let problems prevent you from enjoying sex after age 60. There are many things you can do to make yourself feel better.

Stress can be a huge factor that affects enjoying sex. Some women that are older find that they have things taking place in their life that overwhelm them. Dealing with that stress is very important though to help move on from it. Talking to friends or a professional counselor can certainly be helpful.

A change of partners can be difficult for women as well. Most women are very loyal to their partner and so it can be hard to become intimate with someone else. They may have gotten divorced later in life and just now came back onto the dating scene. Some women have lost their spouse due to death. After being with the same person for decades it is certainly a new experience to have sex with someone different.

Many women will find that it does take longer to become sexually aroused when they are in their 60's. Instead of being frustrated by this a woman just needs to find ways to work with it. Having a relaxing bath with a partner, a nice romantic dinner, or just cuddling for a while can help. A woman needs to make sure her partner understands what will arouse her as well.

The ability to naturally lubricate the vagina can be an issue as well. This is important to address because it can result in sexual stimulation as well as intercourse being painful. There is no reason for a woman to have to deal with this but many suffer in silence. They try to avoid the atmosphere for sex to take place so they don't have to discuss this with their partner.

It is often the result of the vaginal walls becoming thinner as a person gets older. The younger a person is when they go through menopause the more common it is that will occur. Women need to discuss such issues with their gynecologist before they just reach for an over the counter product to assist them with lubrication issues.

Even though women over 60 can end up experiencing some problems, most of them can be overcome. There are very few women who can't end up with a very satisfying sex life as they get older. You may have to work in order to physically and mentally get to that point though. Let your doctor help you too by being willing to share such issues with them. They are professionals so you shouldn't be embarrassed turning to them for assistance.

22- Feel Free to Experiment with Sex even if you are More than 60 Years of Age

There is a great deal of controversy in various societies around the world as to the age when a person should start engaging in sexual intercourse. It can be crazy to know in some cultures it is as young as eleven years old. Others have them waiting until they are in their twenties. What is also strange is that many people have an idea of when they feel someone should stop having sex.

Yet it is important for people to realize that is a very personal decision to make. It is fine to continue having sex into your 60's and beyond. There is no reason to stop doing it simply because of how many birthdays you have compiled over the years. In fact, many individuals in this age group are no where near getting ready to stop. They are enjoying a new found freedom due to retirement and other changes in their lives.

They now have both the time and the desire to experiment with their feelings about their own sexuality. They may finally understand that it is all about what makes them and their partner feel the best. They may feel more relaxed now that they don't have to worry about making a baby. They can just engage in sex for the pure fun and satisfaction that comes with it.

Mentally, a person get themselves into a mode where they never stop to question having sex. They may have really enjoyed it as a younger person and so they continue to do so. It never really crosses their mind that society may see them as being too old to be a part of such activities. People are living longer and healthier lives now than ever before so that is helping to shift the mindset about the topic as well.

For those that aren't as confident as they once were about their own sexual desires, now is the time to do something about it. Work to develop your self esteem by accepting your body for what it is. While it may not be perfect chances are you still have plenty to desire. Make sure your spouse knows you love how their body is too. This is just as important for those over 60 as it is for younger individuals. It is also important for men as well as women.

Having sex when you are over 60 can be a very different experience though. You may feel more relaxed and have more time on your hands for it. You may find you really want to connect with your partner in this way. That means both of you are committed to having a very satisfying sex life.

Feel free to experiment with sex even if you are more than 60 years of age. As long as you are having a great time then that is what matters. If you are struggling with it then see a professional. There can be an array of factors preventing you from having the sex life you long for. Address them now so you can have more time to enjoy a more fulfilling sex life. It doesn't have to stop until you want it to, and for most people that is well beyond the age of 60.

23- Individuals 60 and Older are Very Happy with their Sex Lives

Some individuals feel that getting older isn't going to be very much fun. They believe that everything on their body is going to start to move in directions that aren't very appealing. It is this ideal that they have that makes them think that older individuals much must not take part in having sex. They also believe those that do don't get very much pleasure out of it. Yet they are very wrong in their thinking based on what is really taking place out there.

Most people over the age of 60 are definitely having sex and they are very happy about it. They take part in the activity at least one a week with a regular partner that they have been with for some period of time. They are past the time in their lives when they have to be everything to everyone. It is now time to really focus on their own needs, and that applies to their sexual desires as well.

Some individuals who are over the age of 60 grew up in a very different world. Men were mainly dominant and women were submissive. They stayed at home and took care of the house and the children. Today, there is much more equality among men and women in society. That means women can be more assertive in regards to sexual activities they wish to engage in.

Contrary to popular belief, men really like this. They don't want to be the one to always initiate sexual activities. They want to know they are needed and that they are desired. They want to be sure their partner is having sex because it feels good to them, not just because they feel obligated to keep their partner happy.

Some may think that sex for those over 60 would be boring. After all they should enough experience under their belt to have tried it all. Yet many people in this age group will tell you they are still learning. They are finally following what they wanted to try long ago. Also, as they have gotten older their sexual needs and desires have changed from what they once were.

Communication about sex seems to be more of a standard for people over the age of 60 They feel a connection that goes much deeper now than they did earlier in their lives. While they realize sex isn't what the relationship is all about, it is definitely a very important part of it. They want to become more intimate with their partner and having a great sexual relationship allows that to take place.

For those who have been with the same partner for a very long time, many of the tensions that were once there are gone. With the children grown and retirement in place the struggles over child rearing, money, and even time that were once there aren't anymore. This means that the couple can focus their attention on the needs of each other emotionally and sexually instead of it being consumed by day to day needs.

The sexual behaviors of those over the age of 60 may not be of interest to younger generations. In fact, they find it hard to swallow that their parents or grandparents are taking part in such activities. Yet it should be reassuring to younger generations that such a big part of their life now can continue on as they reach that age themselves down the road before they know it.

While most people you likely know who are over the age of 60 don't go around discussing their sex life in public, you can be sure there is plenty of action still taking place. It is evident from various surveys and questionnaires. The reports from medical offices around the world tell the same story. A great deal of information about those over 60 enjoying sex is also found online where people can share it without disclosing their identity.

24- Are Prescription Medications a good Option For Enjoying Sex when you are in your 60's?

While a person's mind may still want to have a strong and active sex life the body may not always be able to comply. There are some prescription medications out there that have proven to offer those over 60 help with such issues. For example those with diabetes or arthritis may find that they are in too much pain or don't have enough energy for sex.

However, with medication to control their diabetes and a good diet their energy levels increase. There are medications for arthritis too that can prevent the joints from swelling up. This means a person can go about activities including sex and not be in constant pain. It may be something that younger generations take for granted, but when you are physically in pain it can be almost impossible to enjoy the pleasures of sex.

One of the most common types of prescription drugs that men use to help them enjoy sex is Viagra. This is a type of pill that a man takes when he is mentally excited to have sex but the penis isn't getting or maintaining an erection. Many men have found Viagra and similar products have allowed them to have a very enjoyable sex life once again. Their age hasn't been able to stop them from making this important element part of their normal lifestyle.

The pill known as Cialis has also become very popular. This is because a man can take it and then be able to maintain erections when he is ready over the course of the next 36 hours. This means you don't have to plan the act of lovemaking such as you do with Viagra and similar types of prescription medications. It allows the process to be more natural and many men really enjoy having that control over their sexual activities.

There are similar types of prescription medication for women as well. One huge problem for them after menopause is a decrease in the hormone estrogen. As a result they may find they have very little interest in sex. Even if they engage in the act, they just aren't getting the level of pleasure out of it as they once did. Estrogen pills can be prescribed to help a woman gain her libido back.

Prescription medications may be a good option for you if you are older and you really want to improve your sex life. You will need to talk to your doctor about it so a complete assessment can be performed. Identifying the true reasons why you struggle to get an erection or why you aren't enjoying sexual activity is important so be honest with your answers.

There are certainly plenty of prescription medications offered today to help those over 60 be able to continue with a healthy and satisfying sex life. Keep in mind that some of them are a quite expensive though. There are also some side effects associated with each of them to be ready for. You may have to experiment with a variety of different types of prescription medications before you find the one that helps you get to the level of sexual activity you want in your life.

Prescription medications aren't the answer for everyone though. There many be too many health issues for you to consider using them. You may also find that the various side effects also make it difficult for you to enjoy sex. Never use prescription medications for someone else because you are too embarrassed to talk to your doctor about it.

You do owe it to yourself though to see if there is medication that can significantly improve your sex life into your 60's and beyond. There are plenty of people out there in this age group and beyond that find sex more enjoyable now than any other time in their life. Being able to continue engaging in the activity helps to keep them both healthy and happy.

25- Having an Active Sex Life into your 60's can Benefit your Overall Health

Having an active sex life into your 60's can benefit your overall health. There are plenty of statistics to show this can help encourage a person to live a very healthy lifestyle. They will be more concerned about their overall appearance and so they eat better and exercise more.

Many individuals engaging in sex when they are over 60 are also more concerned with their overall health. This means they are willing to keep their appointments for annual check ups. They will also do what the doctor recommends in regards to taking medications and to making changes to their daily habits.

The topic has become more of an issue in our society due to people living longer than ever before. For many people, life doesn't end when they retire as it is only beginning. They find they can pursue new interests and they certainly enjoy having an active sex life. For most people in this age category and older, there is no reason not to continue experimenting with sex and having a great time.

It can be a time to get to know your body in new ways. You may find sex is different at this age though. It may not occur as often and it may not last as long from start to finish. Yet there are still plenty of ways to please your partner to make the most of it. At the same time you can communicate what makes you feel good so you are getting all you can out of the sexual experiences you choose to be a part of.

Having a healthy lifestyle is very important for people of any age. As you get older though it becomes even more important. You can do your part to make sure sexual activity is still a great part of our life when you are in your 60's. Eliminate the use of tobacco and alcohol from your lifestyle. You also want to make sure you eat right, get plenty of rest, and exercise regularly.

Many people in their 60's will tell you that continuing to have sex makes them feel younger than they really are. This carries over into many other aspects of their life as well. They feel better both physically and mentally due to it. They are also able to maintain a very healthy and intimate relationship with someone who is very important to them.

In our society, it has also become more socially acceptable for such behaviors to take place. In the past it was deemed gross or even out of line for people of such age to be thinking about sex. While many of them did, they kept their thoughts on the subject very private. Today they are able to explore them and share them without feeling guilty or feeling like they are being judged.

It is believed that having a positive attitude about sex and realizing that is natural to want to continue having it when you are older plays a vital role in this. Those that don't question their desire to continue having sexual activity into their 60's and later will be able to relax and enjoy it. They aren't going to be inhibited by their age or what is going on around them.

ABOUT THE AUTHOR

Al Fiqi Haytham is a Cairo born criminal lawyer who obtained his Bachelor's Degree in Law from the University of Mansoura in 1997. His is a correspondent and editor for the New Egypt press and is supported by the Supreme Council of the Press. He has also published various legal essays and has acted as an adviser to nursing staff in many different medical   facilities.

In his free time, Al Fiqi Haytham enjoys Play chess ,Playing pool ,Read the legal and scientific books ,Shopping ,Watch foreign movies ,Listening to Beethoven pieces ,Driving. He currently resides in Mansoura with his wife. You can reach him via his blog (http://haythamalfiqi.blogspot.com/) or via email (haythamalfiqi0@gmail.com) to get information about new releases.

CPSIA information can be obtained
at www.ICGtesting.com
Printed in the USA
LVOW13s1955190618
581241LV00028B/880/P